The No Diet

Diet

Victor H. Royer

Updated and revised

The No Diet Diet - Volume 2

Copyright © 2016 by Victor H. Royer.

ISBN-13: 978-1530133093

ISBN-10: 1530133092

Published in the United States of America

GSRHoldingsInc@aol.com

Rev. date: 01/18/2016

The No Diet

Diet

Eat More and Lose Weight!

Victor H. Royer

Published by
GSR Holdings Inc.
Las Vegas

Dedication

With grateful thanks, I dedicate this book to my mother Georgina S. Royer, without whose generous help, vast knowledge, and nutritional skills I would have never been able to write this book.

Table of Contents

Introduction

I weighed 235 lbs. Now I weigh 197 lbs. That's 38 pounds less, and for a man of 5'11" and slight build, that's a lot!

Although I have several academic degrees, here I want to write to you not as an academic, not as some "expert", but just as a plain, normal human being who was simply tired of the rollercoaster ride of weight loss.

I tried the diets, the slim-fasting drinks and shakes, and the rest. What worked for the short-term, didn't work for the long-term. Soon I was back up in weight, fat, unhappy and always tired. I was lugging around so much blubber that I might as well have been carrying a sofa strapped to my back - or so it seemed.

In January, a few years ago, I got really sick. I was very ill, and thought that this was it. Period. I thought my life was over. But, I did get better. And I did it all by myself. I refused to die, or to let myself be that sick ever again. I cured myself, and decided that I was going to do something about the way my life was going. I decided not to be so fat again.

Good decisions, but how to do it?

Good question.

When you think about it, the answer isn't that hard. And no, the answer is not what you may think. The answer is not in the diet pills, it isn't in the diet plans, it isn't in the diet foods, and it isn't even in strenuous exercise.

I still don't do any significant exercise, other than walking a little. I work mostly in front of my computer, as a writer. I basically have a very sedate lifestyle, and all-in-all, the kind of lifestyle I live is the exact opposite of what the medical profession, and the diet proponents, say you must have.

I don't mean to dispute the value of regular exercise, nor the value of properly offered medical assistance, including assistance with dietary supplements, dietary education, and medically-derived dietary assistance.

What I am simply saying, is that the "blueprint" of all these methods does not necessarily work for everyone, nor in the same manner. It certainly didn't work for me.

So, how did I lose 38 lbs in 90 days? And how am I keeping it off? And continuing to lose weight?

Am I starving myself?

No, I am not.

Yesterday, I had a pizza. This morning, I had a marionberry muffin. The day before, two helpings of Chinese food.

I eat what I want, when I want to.

I don't limit how much I eat.

I don't just eat once a day. I eat whenever I feel hungry, and as much as I feel like eating at that moment.

What's the "secret"? Read on – perhaps this will work for you as well as it did for me.

Listen to Your Body

First thing you need to do is listen to your body. To some of you, this may sound like some holistic nonsense. But your body is a fine machine - think of it as a musical instrument ... a band, or an orchestra.

All the various parts working together, one with the other, always in tune. When one part gets out of tune – starts to play badly, off-key, or doesn't play at all - the other parts try to make up for it, like good friends, and pick up the missing beat.

This places a strain on all the other instruments in your body, which now have to work harder and harder. And so more of them start to miss, miss the beat, start to play badly.

In the end, the beautiful song which is your body starts to sound all bad, and the music stops, replaced by noise - and this "noise" is when you start to be sick, be in pain, or start to put on weight.

Your body is simply letting you know that something is wrong, and as a result is trying to find ways to overcome it. If you don't listen to it, it will continue to keep trying to help itself, and keeps sending you the signals.

In the case of weight gain, when the music of your body isn't playing the melody well, it will try to get help - like trying to get more musicians for the band when one or more of the key players are missing, not there, or sick.

The easiest way for this to happen is for you to start to feel more hungry. Your body is asking for replacements for the band, and by adding food, you add more "players" to your body's orchestra, and the song can continue.

However, by doing this, you are adding more and more parts to the band, and therefore the "room" is too small. So, the body expands, adding the room for the extra players.

And so you get fat.

By doing this, you are not helping your body, because you have listened only to the temporary solution to the problem, and not to the cause.

The real problem is that some parts of your body's band have stopped playing, and until you fix those parts, adding more parts will result only in expanding the room necessary to keep all these parts in.

So, in order to get back to the original beautiful melody with which your body started, you need to repair the parts which have gone wrong.

Like on a guitar, when one string breaks, it doesn't matter how well you strum the rest of the strings, the song just won't sound the same.

And neither will your body.

So, the first thing for you to do is try to develop the skills of listening to your body.

These are skills, just like any other skill in life, or work. When you are young, you act on these messages from your body by instinct. But, as you get older, and "wiser", you begin to lose this "instinct", having had it replaced by the conditioning of your life, lifestyle, and social content.

You begin to rely on the "easy fix" - on the pills, prescriptions, diets and so on. Nothing in life is ever easy by itself – it becomes easy with knowledge, and the ability to correctly apply that knowledge.

As a child, you don't have these concerns, because your body and mind are operating together. The "instinct" is the connection between your body and your mind in a way which – at that stage – is the most useful for your survival.

No, this doesn't mean that if you break your arm, or leg, or require surgery for an appendix or hernia, or anything like that, that you should forsake medicine and rely purely on such "instincts".

In all our lives we need to make judgments on when we can help ourselves, and when we need help from others. Here I am speaking only about nutrition and weight gain and weight loss.

A fat child may not necessarily be unhealthy, and neither is this so for all adults.

But for those of us who know that we are fat, and are trying to do something about it, these principles are important.

When you get sick, your body is telling you that something is wrong. However, this is the end of a long line of messages from your body. By the time you get sick, your body has been sending you warning signals for quite some time.

In my case, these warning signals were being given to me for almost the whole year - I just didn't listen. Although I had previously been able to listen, this time I didn't - and I got seriously ill.

What went wrong?

Hard to say – life's pressures, work, business, family, money, future, contentment, society – all these things, and more.

All are contributing factors to these problems, and all cumulatively result in the problems of weight gain.

Alone, a single situation may not be the determining factor –   but put them all together, and, yes, they can be one of the leading contributors to what happened to me - and possibly is happening to you.

Each person is an individual, and as a result no one formula will work for everyone – nor will work exactly in the same manner. That is the primary problem with all these "easy fixes" – such as the diet pills, the diet programs, and so on.

One size does **not** fit all.

Although this should be obvious to most people, the fact is that the companies who market the diet pills, and the diet programs and so on, market them to you as the *only* solution - for *everyone*.

Have you ever bought a pair of shoes which is exactly the same size for everyone in your family? Are all shoes made the same size for all the people in the world? Are clothes made the same size for everyone? Of course not, because we're not all the same. We are individuals. And as a result, no single diet program will always work exactly the same way for everyone.

Therefore, the only way in which a dietary program can work for everyone, is if the individual herself, or himself, customizes the program to her or his body, lifestyle and life.

And to do this can be very simple - if you listen to your body.

How to Listen to Your Body

You already listen to your body without even knowing it. Everyone does this. When you stub your toe, hit yourself with something, get a paper cut, prick yourself with a thorn, or anything like that – it produces pain. This pain is your body talking to you and letting you know that something isn't right.

With pain, we almost always react automatically – we bandage the cut, yell a few words at the chair and the big toe, suck our finger or profess damnation on the instrument, or cause, of the pain. All natural reactions – instinct. Very few people will ever give these situations further thought, nor think about this as a means of communication between your body and your mind.

Often, your mind will even anticipate that something can go wrong if you do it – for example, you're barbecuing, and you know that if you touch the hot grill you'll get burned. Your mind is telling you this, but you still reach for the hot-dog with you fingers and you get burned. Only slightly, thankfully, but you still profess damnation upon the hot-dog, and the grill, suck your finger, wave it about a bit, curse the stars and the universe, and when the pain subsides you go on with your party.

But what did actually happened here?

Here, your mind warned you, but didn't listen. You got burned, and your body told you something was wrong. But did you listen this time? No, you just waved it off and went on with your life.

Yes, this is a simple example, but worth noting. It is the combination of these simple situations which provide the **key** for developing the skills to listen to your body.

While most people will never stop long enough to consciously ponder what happened when you burned you finger on the barbecue – or any such simple "hurt" – these instances are precisely those that allow you to develop skills which are part of you as a human, but which have been educated out of you by your growing-up process, and social conditioning.

In order to recognize this, all you have to do is confront the situation consciously – don't just dismiss it – but think on it. Explain to yourself – aloud if you need to – what happened, and why, and what are the ramifications.

Don't just dismiss the occurrence – but actually take the time to investigate it. Investigate what happened to your body, and how it told you that this was a "hurt".

I realize that to some of you these suggestions may seem odd, or just plain silly.

But they seem this way only because many of us have been educated by our environment into a reliance on external factors, and external assistance, as a solution for everything.

We run to the doctor, but don't ask why. We get the help we need, but don't want to know how it was provided, what it will do to us, or how it works. We just want it to work, and damn how it works, right?

Wrong!

To help yourself, you **must** have some knowledge, some skills, and most of all, a heightened sense of your own self.

Your own self!

You, the individual, are the final frontier.

It is you to whom this is being done, either by yourself, or by others.

If you get external help, what is this going to do to you? After all, it is you who will have to carry on and live with it.

What are the ramifications?

What will this do to you in other circumstances?

I'm sure you know the old story of the surgeon who said the that the operation was a success – but the patient died.

That is as good an example as it gets, and points to the shortcoming of limited thinking.

Yes, the solution may be correct for that one, visible, symptom – but curing it may do more harm than good – unless *the entirety of the individual* is taken into account.

And so it is for weight loss, and so it is for your own powers of decision over your own body.

The examples I gave above of the minor "hurts", are just that – examples. They serve to point out that situations like these, so easily dismissed by most of us, are in actuality the key indicators of how to learn to listen to your own body. By thinking through these minor situations, by examining them, you will begin to have greater control over the information which is being communicated to you by your body on a daily basis.

Fight your body, and your mind may win over it – in the short term – but the ramifications will haunt you for ever.

How many times have you felt sleepy, but didn't lie down?

Perhaps you couldn't, or wouldn't, for whatever reason.

But when you do this, while you may overcome the need – for the moment – it catches up to you eventually. And sometimes much harder than you would ever think.

In fact, that's what we all say – "I didn't do it then, and it's catching up with me".

Right.

That's an indication that you discovered – after the fact – that there was communication happening between your body and your mind, but you didn't listen.

Of course, there are times when we simply can't – but these are *conscious* decisions for very good reasons. We all have these times, and we must handle them when they happen. For most of us, we will eventually have time to recover, and then "get back on track."

But if your goal is to lose weight, there aren't any such excuses. You *always* have to listen to your body – otherwise you are simply lying to yourself and you will not succeed no matter what you do.

Listening to your body means that you become aware of all its functions. No, I don't mean you have to go to medical school and study.

Just be aware.

When you need to go to the restroom, do you give this any thought?

Do you recognize the movements in your body?

Like the "hurt" examples above, these are also the most commonly encountered sequences of communication between your body and your mind, which are virtually always ignored by most of us for what they are. Yes, we act on them, but without thinking. They are common. They happen all the time, and happen by and large regularly.

But just because this happens regularly, it doesn't mean that it is always par for the course.

We all get queasy, have upset tummies, have intestinal problems of one kind or another, and so on.

No, I don't want to get into the implications of loose bowels, but the point is that these situations, like others, are the most commonly encountered and easily learned situations of communications between your body and mind.

By keeping yourself aware of these simple situations, you will learn to become aware of more serious situations, those which are not as easy to recognize, and not as easy to listen to.

Like with everything else in life, the more complex the situation, the harder it becomes to recognize, understand, and act on it.

But once you have learned to listen to your body, and become aware of what it is telling you in the simplest situations, then you will be far more able to listen to the less-prominent circumstances, and therefore be able to act on them for what they *are*, and not just for what they *seem* to be.

And that's how you will be able to come to terms with the information your body is sending you which can result in weight gain, or result in you not being able to keep the weight off.

Weight Gain

If you do too much of anything, it's bad. Water is essential for life, but too much of it and you'll drown. Food is essential for life, but too much of it will kill you. No, this is not the "secret" of this booklet. This is simply a fact. The old story of "Too much of a good thing is bad for you" is true to that extent.

As human beings, we need to eat and drink to survive. This is the "fuel" our bodies need. And our bodies are necessary in order to sustain our minds. Without fuel, we won't continue – we die. But it is the *kind* of fuel we consume which is the determining factor.

Just like in your car – most cars today are configured to run on unleaded gas. But what if you feed it leaded gas? Or a combination of leaded and unleaded? Yes, it will run, but not as well. Continue to do this, and eventually your car will break down. It stops, it won't continue – it dies.

Same applies to different kinds of gasoline for your car – some fuels are low-octane, some middle-octane and some high-octane, all configured for different engines and performance requirements for the kind of car you have.

And the same applies to you, as a human being.

Some of you may require only low-octane food, some need middle-octane food, and some must have high-octane food for optimum performance.

Do you eat for sustenance, or taste? Or both?

Most of us would probably reply that we eat both for sustenance, and for taste. After all, if the food doesn't taste good, it doesn't matter how good it may be for you – it's just a drag to eat it, right?

Oh, yes! I know.

In our society, we as human beings have evolved away from simply seeking food for sustenance, into seeking food which will excite us in the process of eating it.

Taste.

In this regard, we are unique from all of the other mammals on this planet, as indeed we are in many other factors, as a species.

There's nothing wrong with this concept, as long as we recognize it. And listen to our bodies when we get the message to "eat".

Is this message from our body a desire to gratify the taste buds, or a message to say that sustenance is necessary?

When we are hungry, most of us just accept this without any further thought, and we act on it.

Just like when we stub our toe, or burn our finger, or need to go to the potty.

All such actions are derived from messages we receive from our body, but are acted upon without any further conscious thought. And that's where the problems with weight gain arise.

When our bodies send us a message to eat, we "go get something to eat". Something. Usually something which tastes good. Very rarely would I ever hear any of my friends say: "I'm hungry, and I will go eat raw broccoli for maximum sustenance."

Yuck!

So, we get the message to eat, but we don't hear it! We *don't listen* to it, we *just act* on it.

Of course, we want to do things which are pleasant, and therefore eating things which taste good are what we seek out. And no, I am not suggesting that we stop this and instead eat raw broccoli.

Not at all.

The entire point of this book is to show that we do **not** have to do this, and still be able to lose weight – and keep it off.

What contributes to weight gain is not just the volume of foods we consume, and not just which kinds of foods we eat, not even how often we eat, but mostly which *combinations* of foods we eat.

We get fat, and stay fat, because we don't listen to our bodies, and instead of helping the body to "fix" the orchestra, we keep adding more players to it, and therefore have to expand the room to hold all this in.

And so we get big.

No, this doesn't mean that all weight gain is bad – as we get older, our bodies change, and certain parts settle to different areas in larger spaces. This has to do with cellular mechanics, a biotechnical expression for cellular dynamics. Cells have a limited number of divisions (as the facts exist), and as such they will eventually die, and that's how we age. And, as we age, this deterioration in cells contributes to differences in body dynamics, and therefore some parts of us become larger, heavier, and so can our entire bodies.

However, in proportion to our lives, and in proportion to our optimum dimensions, these should be equal, all factors of aging considered.

Therefore, the principles of food and weight loss apply equally well to older people, as to younger adults.

Again, the determining factor is the individual's ability to listen to her or his body as they age, and eat accordingly.

I said above that it is the *kinds* of foods in *combination* which is the overall most important factor which determines whether we get fat, stay fat, or lose weight and keep it off.

And **that's the key**.

See the Food Chart for hints.

Weight Loss

I lost my 38 lbs in 90 days, and I am keeping it off because I listened to my body. I learned to do this by the methods I described above. Now, I want to share with you the factors of food combinations, which are the single key element in weight loss, and continued well-being.

Volume of food is not it.

Neither is frequency of eating.

Not even the kinds of foods you eat.

What *is* the key are the **combinations you eat at the same time**.

Think of the car, and the example of feeding it a combination of leaded and unleaded gas, when the car's engine was designed for unleaded gas. It'll work, but not well. And it won't work for long.

Same applies to your body. For example, eating meat and potatoes – the time-honored staple diet of many people – is quite bad. Not because meat is bad for you, or because potatoes are bad for you. Individually, both foods are necessary for your body.

But put them together, and you get a mess.

Meat contains protein and animal fats, necessary for life. Potatoes contain starch, also necessary for life.

But put the starch together with the animal fats, and you get a paste which is like glue. It is this which contributes to digestion problems, and clogging your arteries. Your body simply cannot process this "glue", along with the "good" proteins, fats, starch and other nutrients, nor can it be completely excreted in the bodily waste.

So, what happens to those parts your body just can't handle?

They get stored.

Like the good machine it is, your body will try to do whatever it can with whatever it is given.

So, it puts this "paste" away in the cells, and there it sits.

And it gets added to, and added to, over and over again – the room needs expansion, and so you get fat.

Your arteries will get clogged. You get sick. You may need major corrective surgery.

Or, you die.

Victor H Royer

And this is only one example.

All food groups are important.

So are the nutritional recommendations by the various medical and nutritional institutions.

But what neither of these groups, nor any of the dietary groups, will tell you is that it is the *combination* of these food groups and nutritional elements which, *when **incorrectly grouped***, will not provide the optimum sustenance nor nutritional benefits.

Simple Guide to Weight Loss

So, what do you do? You have learned to listen to your body. Now, what guidelines do you use to eat the right combinations?

As I've said before, you are an individual. What works for you may not work for your neighbor, husband, wife, friends, or other people.

That's why it is crucial that you decide what works the best for **you**.

When you listen to your body, and listen well, it will tell you. You can then act on that information.

Don't always eat the same things, or the same combinations.

Not only is this boring, but your body has different requirements at different times, seasons, and age.

Seasonal requirements are just as important as nutritional requirements.

In the winter, your body is naturally predisposed to gaining a little weight. It is a natural occurrence, from those eons when the body needed to store weight and fats to assure survival of the being during times of less food.

This is not so for our society anymore, because we have access to any kind of food all year around.

But the instincts are still there.

So, learn this, know this, listen to this, and act accordingly. Just because you gain 5-10 lbs in the winter, don't automatically think you're on your way to being fat, and start some crash diet. Continue with the principles of good eating in correct combinations, and you will do your body well, and it will again set itself back to its optimum weight come spring.

But seasonal changes are not the only factor.

Lifestyle, life, work, stress, and all the other situations all also contribute to weight gain.

When we are stressed, for example, we tend to eat more. Often, we forget to listen to our bodies, and wind up eating the wrong combinations.

And, we get fat.

That's a problem, but it can be easily overcome once we recognize this, and get back to the right track.

Food combinations do not have to taste bad.

If you like steak, eat it with vegetables.

If you like potatoes, eat them without meat.

You can even eat steak and fries, but not regularly because that's a mistake.

However, if you are well on your way toward losing weight by combining foods well, why not eat steak and fries every now and then?

It won't damage this "diet" – because this isn't a diet at all.

It is simply a principle of eating what your body needs when it needs it, and you'll know this if you learn to listen to it. If your body tells you that steak and fries are what it needs, go for it.

But remember what's happening. If you eat steak and fries, or steak and potatoes, *always*, then you'll overdo it and overload your body's ability to process this and the waste it comes with.

The point is – no food, and no food combination is "bad" for you, as long as you eat it not only in moderation, but specifically in a variety of food combinations.

The "variety" factor is important, because this will not only assure that you are getting the right food, right nutrients in the right combinations, but also that the food will taste good.

Food Combination Chart

Here are a few hints on how you can help yourself lose weight, keep it off, and still eat whatever you want whenever you want it.

As a rule, you can eat any of the following with anything else to which it is connected.

Once you have established this protocol of variety, then you can deviate from it as your body tells you – but you should always remember that deviations are just that ... temporary steps away from the system.

As temporary steps, such deviations won't hurt you as long as they remain temporary.

Once you again forget to listen to your body and go back to doing only that which you have done before, and convert the temporary deviations back into the normal, then you'll be in trouble again.

FOOD	EAT WITH	DON'T EAT WITH
Beef	Vegetables or salads	Potatoes or pasta
Potatoes	OK with poultry or fish (unless fried)	Beef
Pasta	With vegetables or vegetable sauces (a little Parmesan excepted, in moderation)	Not with meat, or cheese
Bread	With lettuce, tomato, cucumber, onion,	Not with ham, or beef OK with poultry and fish
Ham	Vegetables, salads, lettuce, cucumber onion, crackers or veggie-salads	No bread, pasta, eggs, potatoes, fries, or pancakes
Eggs	OK with bread, and salads	No meat, bacon, sausages, pancakes crackers, poultry, or ham
Salads	With anything, low-fat dressing or mayo	Not with oily dressings, or full-fat mayo
Sausages	Vegetables, salads	Not with potatoes, pasta, bread, eggs or pancakes

FOOD	EAT WITH	DON'T EAT WITH
Rice	Best food of all! Goes with everything!	NOT fried rice!
Cottage cheese	OK with almost anything	Not with beef
Bacon	OK with bread, salads, crackers, vegetables	Not with eggs, ham, pasta, potatoes, or pancakes
Pancakes	Alone OK with syrup	No butter, eggs, ham, bacon, or sausages
Chicken	OK with almost anything	NOT fried when eaten with other foods
Fried chicken	OK alone, or with coleslaw, or vegetables	Not with anything else
Turkey	Same as chicken	Not fried
Duck, Goose,	Same as chicken	Not fried, and not too often with fries or potatoes
Poultry	Same as chicken	Not fried
Fish	With almost anything	Not fried
Fried fish	Same as fried chicken	Not with anything else

FOOD	EAT WITH	DON'T EAT WITH
Smoked fish	Almost with anything	Not too often with fries
Cheese	OK with bread, alone, or vegetables	Not with pasta, eggs, meat, or sausages
Butter	OK with vegetables	Not with meat or bread
Cooking Oil	OK with vegetables, (vegetable, corn, olive)	Not with meats – use oils sparingly
Fries	OK alone, or with, fish or vegetables, or poultry	Not with beef, fried fish or fried poultry
Corn	With anything	Use butter only if no beef with it
Potato Salad	OK alone, with fish, chicken, turkey, pork, low-fat mayo or dressing	Not with beef or ham
Pasta Salad	OK with almost everything	Not too often with beef or ham.

This Food Chart represents the most widely used foods. Adapt this list for whatever your particular eating habits are, keeping in mind any possible conflicting combinations of foods.

How Long?

How long before you lose weight? That depends on how large you are now, what weight loss you are trying to achieve, what your optimum weight is, or should be, and how skilled and dedicated you will be initially in learning to listen to your body.

When you start a lifestyle change such as I am suggesting, it may take a while. Changes like this will take time, particularly if your body has been abused all your life by not doing what I have here suggested.

I know.

This happened to me as well.

In my case, my body reacted quite quickly. This may not be so for you, or it may be even faster than that.

The point is that if you make a lifestyle change like this, you have to give your body time enough to get used to it, and time enough to allow your body to get rid off all the accumulated waste.

What Else?

Drink a lot of water. Pure water, bottled preferably. Not tap water, in most major cities. Non-chlorinated bottled drinking water is the best. It will help flush out the toxins accumulated in your body.

Stay away from sodas and beer.

Try seltzer instead. If you must have sodas or beer, then only drink them in moderation – no more than two per week for sodas, or two beers per day.

And with beer, try to stay away from American domestic mass-produced beers, because they are 38% sugar!

Drink custom beers, micro-beers, or imported beers like Pilsner Urquell, Heineken, Fosters, Guinness, and so on.

And if you drink more sodas or beer in any one day, prorate it for the rest of the week, and stay off it until you get this sequence back into proportion again.

If you overdo this, you will destroy the benefits you gained elsewhere. Remember, it's all connected.

Drink tea, rather than coffee. Tea has natural anti-oxidants – the same kind found in red wine and grape juice, and is very good for your overall well-being.

But if you can't stand tea, then drink *weaker* coffee, and no more than three cups per day. Use 0% milk as a whitener, instead of cream or artificial whiteners or creamers.

Milk – good for you, but drink only 0% milk. It tastes good, and will provide you with what your body needs, and do so with no-fat.

Sugar – use fructose sugar instead of cane sugar. Fructose sugar comes from fruit, and is far more easily digested by your body than anything else. However, there are differences in which kinds of fructose are better for you. Some aren't, while other are. Which ones?

Those that come "clean" from fruit, and not from artificially-processed plants. You can easily find this out from the labels on the box or packet in which they come. It's better to use cane sugar than those "processed" plant-based fructose substitutes.

And stay away from ALL artificial sweeteners of any and all kinds !! Period!
This especially includes the so-called "diet" drinks, like sodas.

These are chemicals, and your body will

NOT gain the benefit from them in the long run.

Wine – two glasses per day. Drink red, rather than white. Don't drink sparkling wine that much. Go for the more "premium" brands – they are made better, and aren't "sweetened" by use of huge quantities of sugar dumped into the bottling mix.

Popcorn – rarely, but try natural butter flavor. Better this than the "artificial butter" flavors, which are chemicals.

Weight Fluctuation

I also want to remind you that some fluctuations in weight are inevitable, and natural. So, if you are nearing your optimum weight, and suddenly start to see yourself gaining a few pounds, don't despair.

Like seasonal variances, some such situations of intermittent weight gain won't hurt you – unless you have abused your system.

If you didn't abuse yourself, then these minor fluctuations are just a part of your body's system adjusting itself, and the few pounds will go away again.

Vegetarianism or Veganism

Here I am offering a personal commentary, which is simply my opinion. I don't think that pure vegetarianism, or veganism, are the answer.

Like with everything else, all foods are connected, and your body needs them all.

In proper proportions and combinations, as I have said.

Trying to entirely eliminate certain important food groups from your diet will not result in any significant benefits, although some people think so.

For those who are, or want to be, vegetarians, or vegans, I wish you good luck.

I have no problem with that lifestyle. All I wish to point out is that all foods are important in the correct combinations.

All things are connected.

Your body will tell you what it needs and when, if you learn to listen to it, recognize what is being asked, and do accordingly.

And that, dear friends is the end of fat!

Now that we are all thin and healthy, my next book is all about: "Stay Young and Cure Wrinkles." Coming soon.

Now sit an enjoy all the food you want to eat. It's not a sin – and if you do it like I said, you'll still be thin when you've had your fill.

The Joy of Sex!

I thought this would get your attention ☺

And for good reason, of course. It's a well-known fact that having sex burns more calories and unwanted body fats than many other forms of exercise – especially if you have a partner! Solo performances are about half-as-good.

So – why am I telling you this?

Because when dealing with food, nutrition, and the balance of your body – as we have been throughout this book – there's still one more component: Lifestyle.

But "lifestyle" is a boring subject – so it's a lot more fun to call it: The Joy of Sex.

And just like sex, lifestyle is a work in progress. And it evolves as you go on. And as you get older.

At the beginning, it's all about the passion! The pleasure, the experiences, the bonding, the excitement.

It's like that with food, and with your life, and so on.

When it's all new, it's exciting! But as you get used to it, it becomes more routing. And then, later, it can even become a drag. It's kind of like the same old same old. Blahh.

But that's when you need to listen up!

Just as it is important to listen to your body – as I have described in this book – it is likewise important to listen to your lifestyle. By that I mean be *aware* or it more, and more often.

When you start to feel yourself falling into the rut of thinking everything is "always the same", or that "every day is just another day of the same things" – that's the time to perk up, and listen!

It's now that you are beginning to hear the voice of both your body and your mind – particularly your subconscious. Yes, that old thing. Headshrinkers will tell you that more often than not, and charge you $500 for an hour of sleeping on their couch in the process.

But you can resolve all this yourself – and without the cost, or the annoyance of fighting traffic just to go and have your head shrunk.

When you're starting to feel tired – like, say, after lunch, and in the early afternoon – you can perk yourself up in several ways. For example, brush your teeth. The strong minty taste of the toothpaste, and the warm water, and the massaging action of the toothbrush, will do wonders for you! You'll wake up almost immediately, refreshed, happy, and ready to go for the rest of your day.

Or, you can splash yourself with cold water, even in winter, and then some cologne, after-shave, or – for you ladies – some perfume (but different from the one you usually wear, for the scent-difference, which is here the important factor).

Yes, these are only a couple of simple examples, but they are good indicators of what can, and will, help you in your lifestyle, overall.

When you start to feel like your life is in a rut, or feel the loss of excitement, splash some "new" in it. Like the example of brushing your teeth to wake yourself up after lunch, give your lifestyle a "brush-up." Do something different.

Rent a sports car, and go to the track and race around at high speed. It will boost your adrenaline, and change your outlook on your life in many ways! Or, get a cowboy hat and boots, and check yourself out – and surprise your lady in the bedroom!

For ladies, treat yourself to a massage, a spa, a new hairstyle – even if just for the day.

Or, get some of your friends together, and go to a singles night-out, without your present husband, boyfriend, or significant other. Or, get some of those crazy under-things that you see your man drooling over each time the catalogue comes in the mail – or on the computer – and surprise him one night with the fantasy he's always had, but never dared to ask for.

And so on.

The point is this: If you aren't aware that your life needs a re-boot – how can you even try?

And that's also the point – many people just don't know.

Why?

Because they have never learned to listen to their bodies, their minds, or be aware of their "present".

Most of us always live either in the past – good memories and bad – or in the future, such as having to do this, or that, plan for this or that, go there, do this, have to … and so on.

It's life.

For all of us.

As the saying goes: Stop and smell the roses, once in a while.

In the words of the immortal Lilly Tomlin: "The trouble with the Rat Race is: Even if you win, you're still a Rat!"

So, learn to listen, and stop being a Rat!

Your life will thank you for it.

And so will your spouse, significant other, and the rest of the people you know.

And it all starts with listening to your lifestyle, as well as your body.

So, tonight, have some great sex!

And then do it again – differently – and apply the difference to the rest of your life as well.

And THAT is the real Joy of Sex!

Living life YOUR way!

~ Bye now ... ☺

Also by the Author

Casino Magazine's Play Smart and Win
(Simon & Schuster/Fireside, 1994)
Casino Games Made Easy
(Premier, 1999)
Powerful Profits from Blackjack
(Kensington, 2003)
Powerful Profits from Slots
(Kensington, 2003)
Casino GambleTalk: The Language of Gambling and New Casino Games
(Kensington, 2003)
Powerful Profits from Craps
(Kensington, 2003)
Powerful Profits from Video Poker
(Kensington, 2003)
Powerful Profits: Winning Strategies for Casino Games
(Kensington, 2004)
Powerful Profits from Keno
(Kensington, 2004)
Powerful Profits from Casino Table Games
(Kensington, 2004)
Powerful Profits from Internet Gambling
(Kensington, 2005)
Powerful Profits from Video Slots
(Kensington, 2004)
Powerful Profits from Poker
(Kensington, 2005)
Powerful Profits from Internet Poker
(Kensington, 2006)
Powerful Profits from Tournament Poker
(Kensington, 2007)
New Casino Slots (2012)

*Tournament Poker for 21ˢᵗ Century Casinos and the
Internet* (2012)
Eat More and Lose Weight: The No-Diet Diet
(eBook, 2014)
Powerful Profits from Blackjack
(eBook, 2014)
Powerful Profits from Slots
(eBook, 2014)
*Casino GambleTalk: The Language of Gambling and
New Casino Games*
(eBook, 20014)
Powerful Profits from Craps
(eBook, 2014)
Powerful Profits from Video Poker
(eBook, 2014)
Powerful Profits: Winning Strategies for Casino Games
(eBook, 2014)
Powerful Profits from Keno
(eBook, 2014)
Powerful Profits from Casino Table Games
(eBook, 2014)
Powerful Profits from Internet Gambling
(eBook, 2013)
Powerful Profits from Video Slots
(eBook, 2014)
Powerful Profits from Poker
(eBook, 2014)
Powerful Profits from Internet Poker
(eBook, 2014)
Powerful Profits from Tournament Poker
(eBook, 2014)
Great Gamblers: True Stories and Amazing Facts
(Paperback and eBook 2014)

Another Day
(Paperback and eBook 2014)

Riders on the Wind
(eBook 2014)
Great Casino Slots – Volume 1
(eBook 2014)
Great Casino Slots – Volume 2
(eBook 2015)
Casino Secrets – Volume 1
(eBook 2016)
Casino Secrets – Volume 1
(Paperback 2016)
Great Casino Slots – Volume 3
(eBook 2016)
The No Diet Diet – Volume 2
(Paperback 2016)

About the Author

Victor H. Royer, known as Vegas Vic, is the author of 47 books. Mostly known for books, articles, and columns on casino games and gambling, he is also the author of *Great Casino Slots, New Casino Slots, Great Gamblers: True Stories and Amazing Facts*, as well as several titles of fiction, including the western *Riders on the Wind*, and the action romance *Another Day*. Versatile and multitalented, Royer is the creator, producer, and host of the Web-TV shows *"Great Casino Slots"* and *"Casino Secrets"*, now showing at www.LasVegasLiveTV.com

For more information, please visit him at www.MoreCasinoDeals.com.
Sign up for the Insider Advantage Newsletter at: http://www.accessvegas.com/membershipvr